Disability in U.S. Presidents

Report, Recommendations and Commentaries by the Working Group

Bowman Gray Scientific Press, Medical Center Boulevard, Winston-Salem, NC 27157

Printed in the United States of America
ISBN 0-9644070-1-9

DISABILITY IN U.S. PRESIDENTS REPORT, RECOMMENDATIONS AND COMMENTARIES BY THE WORKING GROUP

CONVENERS:

James F. Toole, M.D., LL.B.
Stroke Research Center
& Department of Neurology

Arthur S. Link, Ph.D.
Historian of The Medical Center

The Bowman Gray
School of Medicine,
Wake Forest University

ADMINISTRATION:

Ms. Dianne C. Vernon
Administratrix
Stroke Research Center

Department of Neurology
The Bowman Gray School of Medicine
Medical Center Boulevard
Winston-Salem, NC 27157-1068

Telephone: (910) 716-6103
Fax: (910) 716-5477
Email: jtoole@bgsm.edu

TABLE OF CONTENTS

BACKGROUND AND INTRODUCTION

If the President of the United States must decide within minutes how to respond to a dire emergency, its citizens expect him or her to be mentally competent and to act wisely. Because the presidency of the United States is now the world's most powerful office, should its incumbent become even temporarily unable to exercise good judgment, the consequences for the world could be unimaginably far reaching.

At the Philadelphia convention in May 1787, the framers of the United States Constitution provided, in Article II, Section I:

> ***"In Case of the Removal of the President from Office, or of his Death, Resignation, or Inability to discharge the Powers and Duties of the said Office, the Same shall devolve on the Vice-President, and the Congress may by Law provide for the Case of Removal, Death, Resignation or Inability, both of the President and Vice-President, declaring what Officer shall then act as President, and such Officer shall act accordingly, until the Disability be removed, or a President shall be elected."***

While authorizing Congress to determine the sequence of presidential succession, the framers failed to provide for the orderly transfer of power in the event of inability of the President to discharge duties or, in a more tragic circumstance, if the President is unable to recognize his or her incapacity because of a brain disorder.

The question of the temporary exercise of the executive power first arose on July 2, 1881, when a demented assassin shot President James Abram Garfield, who lingered incapacitated in the presidency until his death on September 18, 1881. Fortunately, there were no important domestic or international problems that had to be addressed, and nothing was done to provide for the temporary assumption of power by Vice-President Chester B. Arthur.

The problem recurred when President Thomas Woodrow Wilson sustained several "small strokes" while at the Paris Peace Conference during the early months of 1919. Physicians cared for his illness, but he continued to represent the United States even though his thinking was impaired. Much worse was the stroke on October 2, 1919, that paralyzed his left side and impaired him until his death on February 3, 1924. Secretary of State Robert Lansing tried to persuade the Cabinet to make Vice-President Thomas R. Marshall the Acting President, but he garnered support neither in the Cabinet nor the Congress. Wilson's months of inability were among the most important in American history because the Treaty of Versailles between Germany and the United States and its allies was before the Senate. A healthy Wilson would probably have obtained the support of many Republican senators, and hence American approval of the Treaty, by agreeing to include a number of relatively innocuous Republican modifications in the articles of ratification. But the stricken President could not defend or promote his position nor would he compromise with even pro-League Republicans. Therefore, ratification that would have brought with it American membership in the new League of Nations was defeated.

A similar situation occurred during the latter years of the incumbency of Franklin Delano Roosevelt. Stricken by poliomyelitis in 1921 and thereafter unable to walk, Roosevelt was impaired but able to serve in office. As Commander in Chief of the United States military, he met the challenges of the dictators of Germany and Italy and of the Japanese militarists. He had overall responsibility for a global war while suffering the complications of uncontrolled severe hypertension. He almost ignored medical advice, and by the time of his fourth election in 1944, Roosevelt was in the very late stages of heart failure and cerebral vascular disease. There is considerable controversy about the degree to which these disorders affected Roosevelt's reluctance to "stand up" to Stalin at the Yalta Conference of February 4 - 11, 1945. However, there is general agreement that dementia affected Roosevelt's refusal to join British Prime Minister Winston Churchill in a military operation to occupy Berlin and Czechoslovakia in advance of the Russians during the last months of the war in Europe. Roosevelt died of hypertensive cerebral hemorrhage soon thereafter, on April 12, 1945.

With global deployment of nuclear weapons following World War II, the possibility that impulsive misjudgment could precipitate a catastrophic disaster increased exponentially. Harry S. Truman was in the pink of health during his incumbency, 1945 - 1953. He and his able Secretaries of State rallied the non-Communist nations in erecting a strong and effective barrier against Soviet expansion in Europe and East Asia. However Truman's successor, Dwight David Eisenhower, suffered several serious illnesses, and his Secretary of State, John Foster Dulles, remained in office while dying of cancer.

Eisenhower, after suffering a heart attack in 1955, intestinal blockage and surgery in 1956, and a stroke in 1957, wrote:

> ***"Three illnesses in three years, any one of which could have been completely disabling if not fatal, convinced me that I should make some specific arrangements for the Vice-President to succeed to my office if I should incur a disability that precluded proper performance of duty over any period of significant length."*** [1]

Acknowledging that even the most short-lived lapse in the President's ability to exercise the executive power is dangerous to the nation, President Lyndon Baines Johnson said in a special message to Congress on January 28, 1965:

> ***"A nation bearing the responsibilities we are privileged to bear for our own security, and the security of the world, cannot justify the appalling gamble of entrusting its security to the immobilized hands or uncomprehending mind of a Commander-in-Chief to command."***

Our nation's awareness of executive vulnerability increased exponentially thereafter. One result was the successful effort by Senator Birch Bayh to achieve congressional approval of the Twenty-fifth Amendment in 1965 and ratification by the necessary thirty-eight state legislatures on February 10, 1967.

---

[1]**(D.D. Eisenhower, The White House Years, II, 227.)**

Sections I and II of the amendment deal with succession. They give the President authority to fill the office of Vice-President, after Congressional approval, when that office is vacated either by a succession to the Presidency or by the elected Vice-President's becoming unable to continue in office because of death, resignation, or removal. No implementing legislation is necessary, as was proved by the appointment of Gerald Rudolph Ford, Jr., and Nelson Aldrich Rockefeller to the vice-presidency in 1973 and 1974, respectively.

Sections III and IV are designed to maintain an active and empowered Chief Executive office if the President is so physically or mentally impaired that his or her advisers judge him or her to be unable to exercise its duties. However, its application has a potential Achilles' heel in the medical evaluations utilized for determining the President's incapacity. Therefore its use may require guidelines established by enabling legislation or Executive Orders.

The Miller Center Commission on presidential disability and the Twenty-fifth Amendment wrestled with the problem of the roles that the physician to the President and consultants should play in determining disability. However, after considering various options, their report[2] concluded:

> ***"The Commission believes that the 25th Amendment provides the means of insuring that the powers and duties of the presidency are always in the hands of one able to perform them. And the Commission believes that this Amendment must be utilized whenever necessary as a normal ingredient in the governmental process."***

---

[2]White Burkett Miller Center of Public Affairs at the University of Virginia and University Press of America, Report of the Miller Center Commission on Presidential Disability and the Twenty-fifth Amendment (1988), p. 23; italics added.

James F. Toole, neurologist, and Arthur S. Link, Ph.D., biographer of Woodrow Wilson, editor of his papers, and longtime professor of history at Northwestern and Princeton Universities, both of whom are now at the Wake Forest University Medical Center, first collaborated in the 1970s in studying the effects of Wilson's strokes on his Presidency.

Later on, in response to an invitation by President Jimmy Carter to the American Academy of Neurology in May 1994, they established the Working Group on Presidential Disability. Toole and Link invited approximately fifty neurologists, internists, historians, political scientists, psychiatrists and psychologists, journalists, and men and women involved in political affairs to meet at the Carter Center in Atlanta in January 26 - 28, 1995, to begin in-depth discussions of problems of presidential disability. During it, Link asserted that physicians should be more forthcoming in offering guidelines and ways and means to evaluate disability, particularly of Presidents.

The group authorized appointment of committees to address special aspects of the Twenty-fifth Amendment. A second conference at Wake Forest University was favored by an address and participation by former President Gerald R. Ford. This conference also included a public forum during which the working group invited input. The final deliberations were held at the White House Conference Center on December 1 - 3, 1996, where the recommendations based on previous

discussions were debated, crystallized, and nine recommendations overwhelmingly adopted. They are presented here along with accompanying commentaries and minority views.

These, it should be said, are based on controlling assumptions, to wit:

1. Many Presidents have experienced health crises which drastically impaired their ability to confront and solve important problems through intelligent consideration.

2. The Twenty-fifth Amendment gives sufficient power to the executive and legislative branches to enable them to act in cases of inability of the President, particularly when disease prevents the President from recognizing the seriousness of the deficit.

3. There should be a contingency plan, approved by the President-elect and Vice-President-elect, stipulating what will be done if any disabling impairment occurs during his or her administration.

4. Medical advice must be sought on a continuing basis for evaluating the President's health and degree of impairment, if any.

5. There must be clear identification of the medical physician who will serve the President as his or her personal physician, and who will be the adviser to the officers designated by the Twenty-fifth Amendment to determine the ability of the Chief Executive to fulfill the duties of his or her office.

The committees that studied particular issues presented their views to the Working Group. The subjects of these eight reports and their committee members are listed on page 34 of this document and will be published along with the full discussions regarding them in the transactions of our three workshops. Participants in the White House conference were given the opportunity to write the minority views which are printed as appendices beginning on page 20.

For recommendation VI concerning the Senior Physician in the White House, a committee of former and current military physicians assigned to the White House offered their experience regarding the profile and title of the recommended physicians office as Appendix II on page 22.

The Working Group recognized that the issues it was considering are of major importance, and that the ideal use of the Twenty-fifth Amendment will come only when the public is well-informed about its purpose and utility. The Working Group offers these recommendations in the hope that they, the commentaries, and minority opinions will be studied and discussed in many forums - schools, civic groups, and perhaps Congressional hearings. Additional materials generated by the Working Group are available in The Wake Forest Law Review (XXX.3, Fall 1995).

This work is a joint effort by volunteers who believe in the need to address a problem of national and international importance. As our population ages, the elderly may begin to fail in their cognitive function long before their physical being is similarly reduced. This leads to the dichotomy of healthy physique but impaired cognition which is not always apparent. This problem occurs at all

levels of society, including local, corporate, national, and international arenas. People with failing minds who are in positions of responsibility may make faulty judgements without their cognitive disorder being recognized. Serious consequences can result and cause enormous and widespread effects which could be avoided if mechanisms to identify cognitive decline had been in place.

If the time comes - as surely it shall - when the Twenty-fifth Amendment must be used, an informed nation will evaluate its leaders by how well they use it for the good of the country.

James F. Toole, M.D., Arthur S. Link, Ph.D., and J. Howell Smith, Ph.D.
Editors for this Publication

Winston-Salem, N.C.
June 1997

EDITORIAL COMMITTEE FOR TRANSACTIONS

RECOMMENDATION ONE

The Twenty-fifth Amendment is a powerful instrument which delineates the circumstances and methods for succession and transfer of the power of the Presidency. It does not require revision or augmentation by another constitutional amendment. However, guidelines are needed to ensure its effective implementation.

COMMENTARY

Since its ratification in 1967, the Twenty-fifth Amendment to the United States Constitution has enhanced America's ability to respond to presidential inability. The Amendment provides constitutional procedures for transferring power, voluntarily or involuntarily, from President to Vice-President. It makes it clear that the Vice-President acts as, but does not become, President during the period of inability and that when the President is able to resume the powers and duties of the office he or she can do so. It removes such constitutional questions as "Who decides when, or if, the President is unable to discharge his or her duties? What is the status of the President and Vice-President during the period of the inability? Could the President later resume office?" which before 1967 inhibited those responsible from appropriate transfers of presidential power. Moreover, by designating the Cabinet to act along with the Vice-President as constitutional decision-makers, it increases the likelihood that Vice-Presidents would act, when appropriate, by assuring the President's political associates against usurpation of the President's office while at the same time, protecting the Vice-President from criticism. By providing that Congress would resolve any dispute between the Vice-President and Cabinet on the one hand and the President on the other, it imposes a further check on improvident behavior while providing a mechanism for resolution by politically accountable individuals. Finally, by allowing Congress the option to substitute "such other body as Congress may by law provide" for the Cabinet, the Amendment affords a means by which to change that feature in the light of experience.

Although its authors and the Working Group viewed the amendment as imperfect, revision or augmentation by amendment appears to be impractical and might create greater problems than it sought to correct.

RECOMMENDATION TWO

The Twenty-fifth Amendment has not been invoked in some circumstances envisioned by its founders. When substantial concern about the ability of the President to discharge the powers and duties of office arise, transfer of power under provisions of the Twenty-fifth Amendment should be considered.

COMMENTARY

The Amendment provides a mechanism for transferring presidential power whenever appropriate constitutional decision-makers determine that the President "is unable to discharge the powers and duties of his office." The framers of the Amendment intended to address a wide range of situations involving temporary or permanent physical or mental illness which could prevent the President from exercising his or her powers and duties when public business requires Presidential leadership.

During President Reagan's term of office there were occasions when the provisions of the Twenty-fifth Amendment might have been used. Following the assassination attempt on March 30, 1981, President Reagan underwent surgery under general anesthesia and, thereafter, was seriously ill during parts of his convalescence. Apparently no one suggested that the President invoke Section 3 when he could have, and suggestions that the appropriate decision-makers invoke Section 4 were dismissed.

When President Reagan underwent colon surgery in July 1985, he transferred powers to Vice-President Bush. Some regard this occasion as its first use, because he followed the stipulations of Section 3.

During the Bush Administration, consideration was given to invoking Section 3 in May 1991 when the President developed irregular heartbeat (atrial fibrillation). The problem was resolved without general anesthesia or other disability and, accordingly, the amendment was not invoked.

RECOMMENDATION THREE

A formal contingency plan for the implementation of the amendment should be in place before the inauguration of every President.

COMMENTARY

Documented guidelines are needed to insure the consistent application of the Twenty-fifth Amendment in appropriate situations. This can best be accomplished by a White House contingency plan which clearly delineates alterations of function, including cognitive, judgmental, behavioral, and communicative capacities, which should cause consideration of a transfer of power. It must define precise lines of authority and communication and specify exact procedures for its execution. It should also include detailed instructions for specific procedures and lines of communication to be followed for implementing the provisions of Sections 3 and 4, respectively.

The contingency plan must be developed during the transition period and implemented at the time of inauguration. Every aspect should personally be approved by the President, be clearly understood by the President's spouse, the Vice-President, and all government officials and staff members who would be involved in its implementation. The plan should state explicitly that it constitutes an order by the President for specific actions to be taken in case of Presidential inability to carry out the duties of office.

Furthermore, the plan should delineate those situations and medical conditions which would normally warrant a voluntary transfer of power under the provisions of Section 3 or an involuntary transfer of power under the provisions of Section 4. Approval of the plan by the President would constitute authorization for the release of all medical information to the Vice-President and principal officers of the executive departments in any situation where an involuntary transfer of power must be considered.

The contingency plan pertaining to presidential inability and continuity of government will contain highly sensitive information and should be classified. Nevertheless, an unclassified summary of the contingency plan, including its medical aspects, should be released to the public at the beginning of each presidential term.

RECOMMENDATION FOUR

Determination of presidential impairment is a medical judgment based upon evaluation and tests. Close associates, family, and consultants can provide valuable information which contribute to this medical judgment.

COMMENTARY

The assessment of impairment is a medical responsibility. The Physician to the President is responsible, with the assistance of appropriate medical and non-medical consultants, for determining and documenting the extent to which impairment might affect the cognition, judgment, behavior and communication abilities of the President. The Physician to the President should communicate and interpret these findings to the constitutionally designated decision-makers responsible for determining presidential inability under the provisions of the Twenty-fifth Amendment.

While the determination of presidential inability is to be made by constitutionally empowered officials, conclusions concerning the degree of medical impairment should significantly inform their judgment. Some medical conditions, such as coma, severe dementia, massive trauma, general anesthesia for major surgery, major psychiatric disorders, and terminal cancer produce impairment of such severe degree as always to warrant consideration of invoking the 25th Amendment.

For minority opinion see Appendix I on page 20.

RECOMMENDATION FIVE

The determination of presidential inability is a political judgment to be made by constitutional officials.

COMMENTARY

Working Group consensus was achieved by consideration of the following:

1. Drawing a clear distinction between the terms "impairment" and "inability." Judging presidential impairment is a medical determination; certifying presidential inability relates to the powers and duties of the office he or she is unable to execute as a consequence of that impairment.

2. Determining impairment should rest solely with the Senior Physician in the White House and consulting medical specialists. Declaring inability pertains to constitutional, administrative, and political considerations as determined voluntarily by the President (Section 3 of the Twenty-fifth Amendment), or by the Vice-President and the principal officers of the executive departments should the President be unable — or unwilling — to do so (Section 4 of the Twenty-fifth Amendment).

3. Issues such as the urgency of executive functions or perceived risks to public interest must be considered before initiating disclosure and discovery procedures for either section.

4. In accordance with each administration's contingency plan, the President should agree that full disclosure of all medical information to the Vice-President and principal officers of the executive departments be made in order to assist in their determination.

RECOMMENDATION SIX

The President should appoint a physician, civil or military, to be Senior Physician in the White House and to assume responsibility for his or her medical care, direct the Military Medical Unit, and be the source of medical disclosure when considering imminent or existing impairment according to the provisions of the Twenty-fifth Amendment.

COMMENTARY

The President must have full authority to choose his or her own physician. This medical doctor will be the focus for medical information about the President and will render personal care to the President as well as collecting all needed medical information about the President's fitness for office. The Senior Physician in the White House must be the person to advise the President, Vice-President, Cabinet, and others stipulated by the Twenty-fifth Amendment when medical evaluation is required.

The Working Group, therefore, believes that it is necessary to create the office of Senior Physician in the White House with clearly delineated responsibility and authority. This Senior Physician must meet the highest professional standards and enjoy the respect and esteem of the medical community.

A committee of military physicians appointed to the White House medical unit provided the Working Group with recommendations concerning the appropriate title and organizational rank for the office.* While the Senior Physician in the White House might be either civilian or military, the office of Senior Physician should be formally separated from, and independent of, the White House Military Office. Whether civilian or military, the Senior Physician must have full military medical support. The Working Group recommends that the office be accorded title and rank of Assistant to the President, Deputy Assistant to the President, or an equivalent military rank. In addition, the Senior Physician may retain additional titles or appointments, such as Senior Physician in the White House Medical Unit, as appropriate.

The current role of physicians assigned by the military branches to duty in the White House should remain in place. It is expected that the Senior Physician in the White House Medical Unit will carry the responsibility of the personal Physician to the President at the times when the office of Senior Physician to the President is vacant.

* Appendix II on page 22.

RECOMMENDATION SEVEN

In evaluating the medical condition of the President, the Senior Physician in the White House should make use of the best consultants in relevant fields.

COMMENTARY

The Working Group recognized that there might be instances when medical consultation would be essential for optimal care and for the development of recommendations by the Senior Physician to the President. The Working Group considered ways for developing consultant(s) resources; on the one hand, an established panel of distinguished consultants could be activated when needed by the Senior Physician in the White House. Alternatively, ad hoc consultants could be selected when need arose, perhaps drawn from a roster of recognized medical specialists.

After lengthy discussion, it was concluded that the best system would result from ad hoc selection of consultants by the Senior Physician in the White House, who must be able to select from any and all consultants appropriate to the specific medical issue(s) at hand.
Considerations included that no one can foresee which experts would be best for a medical crisis. Furthermore, there was concern that appointment to a standing commission could become a political process rather than one of merit.

For minority opinion see Appendix III on page 23.

RECOMMENDATION EIGHT

Balancing the right of the public to be informed regarding Presidential illness with the President's right to confidentiality presents dilemmas. While the Senior Physician to the President is the best source of information about the medical condition of the President, it is the responsibility of the President or designees to make accurate disclosure to the public.

COMMENTARY

Because the President must make critical decisions for the nation, the public must know enough about presidential mental and physical well being to be confident of his or her judgment. The nation is clearly entitled to that information. But Presidents are also patients and are entitled to privacy which cannot be as encompassing as that of ordinary patients. Presidents tend to surround themselves with aides whose loyalty is primarily personal and who, at times, have concealed the gravity of presidential illnesses. The Working Group could not reach unanimity regarding methods for avoiding concealment.

The group acknowledged that even the most confidential evaluation might be made public and raise damaging political questions. This possibility might cause President and aides to evade or thwart the objectives of medical candor and confidentiality that is needed. Furthermore, Presidents might invoke the doctrine of separation of powers and decline to submit to any congressionally-mandated examiners. The dilemma is more easily delineated than solved.

RECOMMENDATION NINE

The Twenty-fifth Amendment provides a remarkably flexible framework for the determination of presidential inability and the implementation of the transfer of powers. Its provisions should be more widely publicized and its use destigmatized.

COMMENTARY

The Presidency of the United States possesses unparalleled authority and power. Both have been guarded zealously by the President and those around him. As a result, there have been times when, unknown to the American people, the Chief Executive was unable to perform the powers and duties of office.

The ratification of the Twenty-fifth Amendment recognized that the national interest demanded an end to this dangerous practice. In two critical sections, the Amendment provides procedures for ensuring that the powers and duties of the Presidency will always reside — permanently or temporarily — with one capable of using them properly.

Section 3 provides for voluntary transfer of power from the President to the Vice-President, who will serve as acting President when the President believes his medical condition will make it impossible for him to perform. It provides that the President can resume his office when he or she recovers. The framers of the Twenty-fifth Amendment believed that Section 3 would encourage Presidents to act voluntarily and responsibly in disclosing and seeking treatment for illnesses. It was their belief that most incidents of presidential inability could be handled in this manner.

Section 4 provides for occurrences in which a President does not, for any reason, declare his or her inability to perform in office. In such circumstances, the Vice-President and a majority of the Cabinet may determine that it is in the national interest for the Vice-President to serve as acting President. If the President regains the ability to perform, he or she may reclaim the Presidency. Here, too, the provisions are specific.

The precedent established by Presidents Bush and Clinton of creating a contingency plan governing all circumstances of presidential inability is indispensable to the implementation of the Twenty-fifth Amendment. It is imperative that senior presidential officials and the presidential spouse know what inability and transition procedures have been approved by the President in advance of any inability. Further, the nation should be apprised of the general parameters of such contingency plans. The news media should have a major role in creating an environment in which the 25th Amendment can and will be implemented. It can help make the public aware of its existence and predispose citizens to insist that it be implemented when appropriate. Those who are given the responsibility for governing must be made to understand that their failure to implement the amendment in case of presidential impairment could put the nation in peril.

APPENDIX I

MINORITY OPINION REGARDING RECOMMENDATION IV
John D. Feerick, J.D., Joel K. Goldstein, J.D. and Senator Birch Bayh

This separate statement expresses our reservations regarding Recommendation IV and some of the commentary discussing "presidential impairment."

We have the following specific concerns. First, the distinction between "presidential impairment" and "presidential inability," is not likely to be understood by the public or media, particularly if not considered in conjunction with Recommendation V.

Second, that there will be a determination of presidential impairment separate from the constitutional determination of presidential inability implies that a two-threshold determination must take place when, in fact, the Constitution speaks of only one. This creates the misleading impression of two "determinations" with equal weight when, in fact, the Constitution stipulates one.

The legislative history and debates of the 25th Amendment leave no doubt that only the constitutional decision-makers, are entrusted with the determination of presidential inability. Integral to that determination is whether there is an impairment of the President that prevents him or her from discharging the powers and duties of office. As Senator Birch Bayh made clear in the Senate debates of February 19, 1965:

> [T]he words "inability" and "unable" as used in [Section 4 of the Amendment] . . . , which refer to an impairment of the President's faculties, mean that he is unable either to make or communicate his decisions as to his own competency to execute the powers and duties of his office. I should like for the RECORD to include that as my definition of the words "inability" and "unable."

The dual track approach contained in recommendations IV and V therefore, is not constitutionally based or wise.

Third, the notion of a "determination of presidential impairment" conveys an inaccurate picture of the proper role of medical advice in decisions under section three and section four of the Twenty-fifth Amendment. Recommendation IV implies that the medical role will be limited to a single "determination"; in fact, in many instances the appropriate doctors will be involved in a less formal but continuing advisory role to the constitutional decision-makers. In many instances, the doctors will not be making a single "determination" but will be offering medical advice and responding to questions on a continuing basis.

Fourth, the implication that there will be a formal "determination" of presidential impairment in addition to the constitutionally required determination of presidential inability raises some concerns regarding the operation of sections three and four. Even information confidential in the While House is likely to leak. We are concerned that a determination that the President was impaired, if leaked, would be seen as a judgment that the President was unable to discharge his duties. This would have the effect either of compromising his ability to lead or of forcing the constitutional decision-makers to a decision they otherwise might not make.

In essence, we believe that the Constitution requires that "[t]he determination of presidential inability is a political judgement to be made by constitutional officials." (Recommendation V) Constitutional decision-makers will generally require medical advice from appropriate medical experts (in accordance with Recommendations VI and VII) regarding the President's condition in making decisions under section three and four as to whether the President is able to discharge the powers and duties of his office. The legislative history surrounding the adoption of the Twenty-fifth Amendment makes clear that its framers intended that constitutional decision-makers would solicit appropriate medical advice. Decisions regarding the exercise of executive power under the Twenty-fifth Amendment, however, should be made by accountable constitutional officials, not by doctors, attorneys or others who have not been elected by the people or confirmed by their representatives.

APPENDIX II

REPORT BY FORMER AND CURRENT MILITARY PHYSICIANS ASSIGNED TO THE WHITE HOUSE REGARDING RECOMMENDATION VI

John E. Hutton, Jr., M.D., Lawrence C. Mohr, M.D., E. Connie Mariano, M.D., and James M. Young, M.D.

1. The President has and will continue to exercise his or her choice of physician to provide health care while he or she occupies the office of President of the United States.

2. It is recommended that the President appoint a Senior Physician to a position as his or her personal physician in the Executive Office of the President.

3. This physician should be the Senior Physician in the White House with responsibility for facilitating the application of the Twenty-fifth Amendment.

4. The Senior Physician in the White House could be designated as Physician to the President, Physician to the White House, or Senior Physician of the White House Medical Unit.

5. It is recommended that the Senior White House Physician be accorded a title such as Assistant to the President or Deputy Assistant to the President, or equivalent military rank.

6. The office of Senior Physician in the White House should be an entity separate from the White House Military Office.

7. Because the Senior White House Physician may be a civilian or military physician, it is recommended that she or he have military medical support.

APPENDIX III

MINORITY OPINION REGARDING RECOMMENDATION VII

Herbert L. Abrams, M.D., Hugh Evans, M.D., Mr. Wayne King

Bert Park, M.D., Jonathan E. Rhoads, M.D., Robert S. Robins, M.D.

1. A majority of the Subcommittee on Public Disclosure believed that the President's physician was subject to such a powerful potential conflict of interest that it was impossible to assure the prevention of cover-ups.

2. The Subcommittee, therefore, recommended the creation of a Consulting Commission on the Health of the President by Congressional resolution or statute.

3. Such a dispassionate group of expert physicians would be available to provide consultative advice and support to the President's physician and to report to the public on the state of the President's health in the event that the question of impairment arose.

4. Because they would not be subject to Presidential pressure, nor serve purely at the President's pleasure, as does the White House physician, they would enhance public confidence, allay suspicions of cover-up, and provide a solid base of medical information for the President, the Vice-President and the Cabinet if invocation of the Twenty-fifth Amendment was under consideration.

THE MEMBERS LISTED BELOW HAVE ENDORSED THESE RECOMMENDATIONS AND COMMENTARIES UNLESS NOTED BY MINORITY OPINIONS

Herbert L. Abrams, M.D. ***
Stephen E. Ambrose, Ph.D. *
George J. Annas, J.D. *
The Honorable Birch Bayh ***
Leonard Berg, M.D. *
Frank Davidoff, M.D. *
David Drachman, M.D. ***
Joseph English, M.D. ***
Hugh E. Evans, M.D. ***
John Feerick, LL.B. **
Joseph J. Fins, M.D. *
Phil Fontanarosa, M.D. ***
The Honorable Gerald R. Ford *
H. Miles Foy, J.D. ***
John A. Gergen, M.D. ***
Robert E. Gilbert, M.D. ***
Joel K. Goldstein, J.D. ***
Murray Goldstein, D.O., M.P.H. *
Lazar J. Greenfield, M.D. *
Katy Harriger, Ph.D. ***
Eugene A. Hildreth, M.D. ***
Steven Hochman, Ph.D. **
Robert J. Joynt, M.D., Ph.D. ***
Mr. Wayne King ***
Francis I. Kittredge, Jr., M.D., J.D. ***
Arthur S. Link, Ph.D. ***
E. Connie Mariano, M.D. ***
Stephen McConnell, Ph.D. *
T. Jock Murray, M.D. **
Adrianne Noe, Ph.D. *
Bert Park, M.D. ***
Jonathan E. Rhoads, M.D. ***
Steven P. Ringel, M.D. *
Daniel Ruge, M.D., Ph.D. **
James Semans, M.D. ***
P. John Seward, M.D. *
J. Howell Smith, Ph.D. ***
James F. Toole, M.D., LL.B. ***
Kenneth M. Viste, Jr., M.D. ***
Robert Walsh, J.D. **
Jack P. Whisnant, M.D. ***
Mr. Thomas G. Wicker **
Jerry M. Wiener, M.D. ***
James M. Young, M.D. *

Workshops in which Participated:

1*
2**
3***

PRESIDENTIAL DISABILITY PARTICIPANTS

THE CARTER CENTER OF EMORY UNIVERSITY — ATLANTA, GA

JANUARY 26-28, 1995

Herbert L. Abrams, M.D.
Stephen E. Ambrose, Ph.D.
The Honorable Birch Bayh
Leonard Berg, M.D.
Douglas Brinkley, Ph.D.
President Jimmy Carter
Kenneth R. Crispell, M.D.
Lloyd N. Cutler, LL.B.
David A. Drachman, M.D.
Joseph T. English, M.D.
Hugh E. Evans, M.D.
Phil B. Fontanarosa, M.D.
Mr. Stephen A. Foster
H. Miles Foy, J.D.
John A. Gergen, M.D.
Robert E. Gilbert, Ph.D.
Joel K. Goldstein, J.D.
John Hardman, M.D.
Katy J. Harriger, Ph.D.
Eugene A. Hildreth, M.D.
Steven H. Hochman, Ph.D.
Robert J. Joynt, M.D., Ph.D.
Mr. Wayne King
Francis I. Kittredge, Jr., M.D., J.D.
Burton J. Lee, III, M.D.
Arthur S. Link, Ph.D.
E. Connie Mariano, M.D.
Stephen McConnell, Ph.D.
Cheryl E. Mills, J.D.
Lawrence C. Mohr, M.D.
T. Jock Murray, M.D.
Richard E. Neustadt, Ph.D.
Bert E. Park, M.D.
Jerrold M. Post, M.D.
Jonathan E. Rhoads, M.D.
Robert S. Robins, Ph.D.
Teresa Wynn Roseborough, J.D.
Daniel Ruge, M.D., Ph.D.
James H. Semans, M.D.
P. John Seward, M.D.
J. Howell Smith, Ph.D.
James F. Toole, M.D., LL.B.
Kenneth M. Viste, Jr., M.D.
Robert K. Walsh, J.D.
Jack P. Whisnant, M.D.
Mr. Thomas G. Wicker
Jerry M. Wiener, M.D.
Frank B. Wood, Ph.D.
Edwin M. Yoder, Jr., D. Litt

Observers

Mr. Robert Conn
William A. Link, Ph.D.
Ms. Jane Nevins
Mr. James O'Sullivan
Robert A. Pastor, Ph.D.
Ms. Barbara Rich
Mr. Wayne Thompson
William W. Toole, J.D.

Guests

Mrs. Kris Fontanarosa
Mrs. Jan Viste
Mrs. Marilyn Abrams
Mrs. Gerry Berg
Mrs. Marge Crispell
Mrs. Jacqueline Gergen
Dr. Katharine Rhoads
Mrs. Marjorie Robins
Mrs. Mary Semans
Mrs. Patricia Toole
Mrs. Patricia Whisnant
Mayor Martha Wood

PRESIDENTIAL DISABILITY PARTICIPANTS

WAKE FOREST UNIVERSITY — WINSTON-SALEM, NC

NOVEMBER 10-12, 1995

Herbert L. Abrams, M.D.
The Honorable Birch Bayh
Kenneth R. Crispell, M.D.
Lloyd N. Cutler, LL.B.
David A. Drachman, M.D.
Joseph T. English, M.D.
Hugh E. Evans, M.D.
John D. Feerick, LL.B.
Phil B. Fontanarosa, M.D.
The Honorable Gerald R. Ford
H. Miles Foy, J.D.
John A. Gergen, M.D.
Robert E. Gilbert, Ph.D.
Joel K. Goldstein, J.D.
Katy J. Harriger, Ph.D.
Eugene A. Hildreth, M.D.
Steven H. Hochman, Ph.D.
John D. Holmfeld, Ph.D.
Robert J. Joynt, M.D., Ph.D.
Mr. Wayne King
Francis I. Kittredge, Jr., M.D., J.D.
Burton J. Lee, III, M.D.
Arthur S. Link, Ph.D.
E. Connie Mariano, M.D.
Lawrence C. Mohr, M.D.
Bert E. Park, M.D.
Jerrold M. Post, M.D.
Jonathan E. Rhoads, M.D.
Robert S. Robins, Ph.D.
Daniel Ruge, M.D., Ph.D.
James H. Semans, M.D.
J. Howell Smith, Ph.D.
Kathy B. Smith, Ph.D.
James F. Toole, M.D., LL.B.
Kenneth M. Viste, Jr., M.D.
Robert K. Walsh, J.D.
Jack P. Whisnant, M.D.
Mr. Thomas G. Wicker
Jerry M. Wiener, M.D.
Frank B. Wood, Ph.D.
Edwin M. Yoder, Jr., D. Litt

Observers

Walter Davis, M.D.
Jack Fleer, Ph.D.
Lt. William McGee, M.S.C., U.S.N.
Kari Murros, M.D.
William W. Toole, J.D.

Guests

Mrs. Marge Crispell
Mrs. Emalie Feerick
Mrs. Jacqueline Gergen
Dr. Katharine Rhoads
Mrs. Mary Semans
Mrs. Jeanette Smith
Mrs. Jane Yoder
Mrs. Patricia Toole

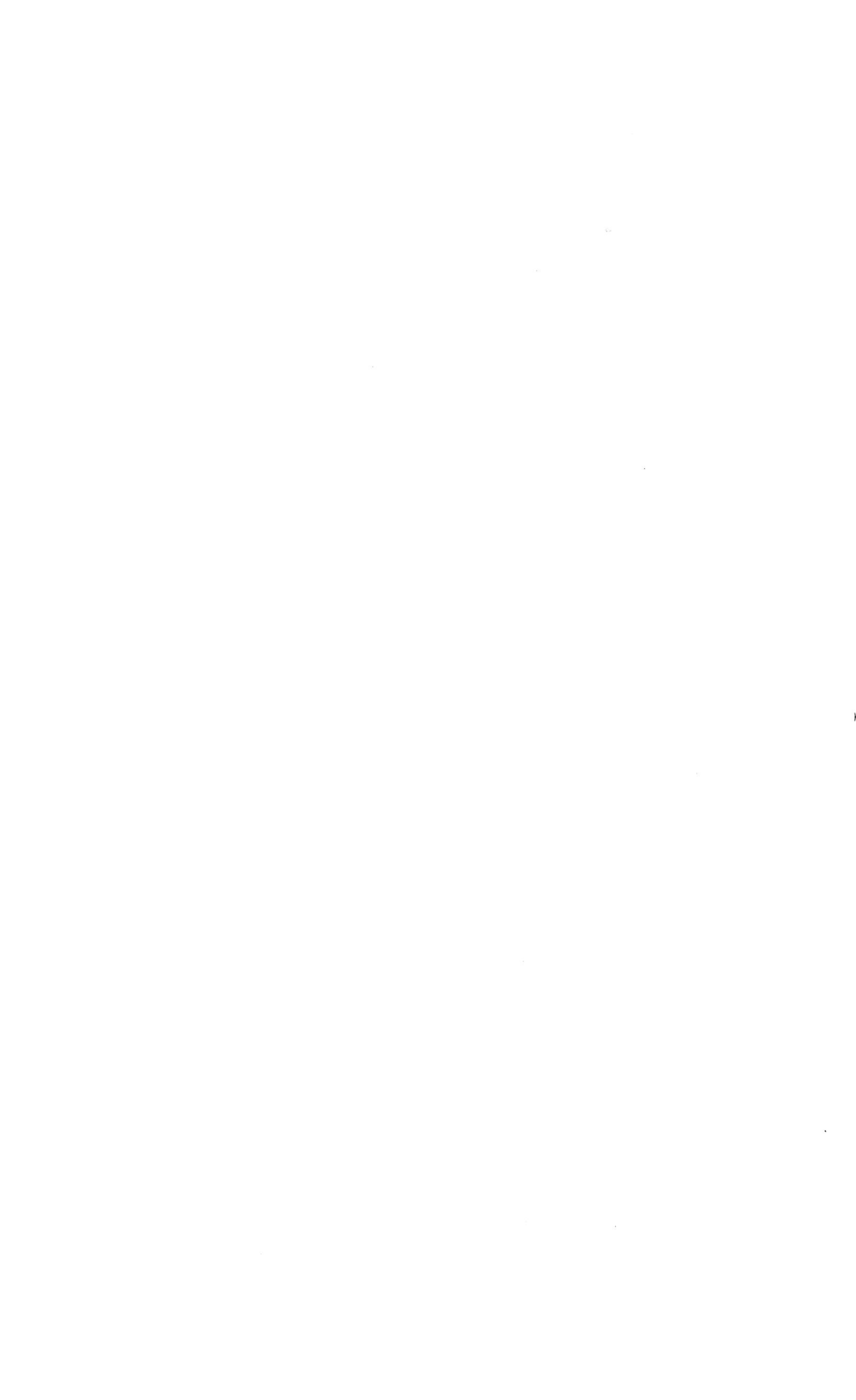

PRESIDENTIAL DISABILITY PARTICIPANTS

THE WHITE HOUSE CONVENTION CENTER — WASHINGTON, DC

DECEMBER 1-3, 1996

Herbert L. Abrams, M.D.
Lawrence Altman, M.D.
George J. Annas, J.D.
The Honorable Birch Bayh
Lloyd N. Cutler, LL.B.
Frank Davidoff, M.D.
David A. Drachman, M.D.
Joseph T. English, M.D.
Hugh E. Evans, M.D.
John D. Feerick, LL.B.
Joseph Fins, M.D.
Phil B. Fontanarosa, M.D.
H. Miles Foy, J.D.
John A. Gergen, M.D.
Robert E. Gilbert, M.D.
Joel K. Goldstein, J.D.
Murray Goldstein, D.O., M.P.H.
Lazar Greenfield, M.D.
Katy J. Harriger, Ph.D.
Eugene A. Hildreth, M.D.
John E. Hutton, Jr., M.D.
Robert J. Joynt, M.D., Ph.D.
Mr. Wayne King
Francis I. Kittredge, Jr., M.D., J.D.
Arthur S. Link, Ph.D.
E. Connie Mariano, M.D.
Lawrence C. Mohr, M.D.
T. Jock Murray, M.D.
Adrianne Noe, Ph.D.
Bert E. Park, M.D.
Jerrold M. Post, M.D.
Jonathan E. Rhoads, M.D.
Steven Ringel, M.D.
Robert S. Robins, Ph.D.
James H. Semans, M.D.
J. Howell Smith, Ph.D.
James F. Toole, M.D., LL.B.
Kenneth M. Viste, Jr., M.D.
Jack P. Whisnant, M.D.
Jerry M. Wiener, M.D.
Frank B. Wood, Ph.D.
Edwin M. Yoder, Jr., D. Litt
James Young, M.D.

Observers

Luther Self, Ph.D.
William W. Toole, J.D.

Guests

Mrs. Marilyn Abrams
Mrs. Ann Davidoff
Mrs. Kris Fontanarosa
Mrs. Jacqueline Gergen
Mrs. Margaret Joynt
Dr. Katharine Rhoads
Mrs. Marjorie Robins
Mrs. Sally Self
Mrs. Jeanette Smith
Mrs. Claudina Toole
Mrs. Patricia Toole

BENEFACTOR AND SPONSORSHIPS

Benefactor

The Charles A. Dana Foundation (1, 2, 3)

Sponsors

Alzheimer's Association (1)
American Academy of Neurology Education & Research Foundation (1, 2, 3)
American Academy of Physical Medicine & Rehabilitation (1)
American Bar Association (2)
American College of Physicians (2, 3)
American College of Surgeons (3)
American Medical Association (1, 2, 3)
American Neurological Association (1, 2, 3)
American Psychiatric Association (1, 2, 3)
Mary Duke Biddle Foundation (2, 3)
The Carter Center (1, 2, 3)
Bert E. Park, M.D. (1, 3)
Wake Forest University (1, 2, 3)
- The Bowman Gray School of Medicine (1, 2, 3)
- Reynolda Campus (1, 2)
- Stroke Research Center (1, 2, 3)

Numbers in parenthesis indicate years of sponsorship:

1995 = 1
1995 = 2
1996 = 3

ACKNOWLEDGEMENTS

The many tasks required for planning and implementing our meetings could not have been carried out successfully without the hard work and cooperation of a large number of talented, dedicated individuals. Foremost among these is Dianne C. Vernon who has coordinated the Stroke Center team effort with staff members Kelley Needham, Sherri Blackwell, Tara Love, Pamela Beck, Janet Hanson, and Ralph Hicks, Jr.

WE ARE ESPECIALLY GRATEFUL TO OUR LIAISONS:

- Lisa Wiley, Eric Oliver and the staff at The Carter Center who graciously responded not only to the needs of the organizers but also to the many requests of our participants.

- Linda Michalski, Melody Graham, Cheryl Walker, Ruth Sartin and Imogene Setliff of the Wake Forest University staff who worked closely with the Bowman Gray Medical Campus in planning and organizing a very successful meeting.

- Connie Mariano, M.D., White House Physician, for the invitation to the White House Conference Center and to Lt. William McGee of the Medical Unit for coordinating local arrangements.

- Dr. Adrianne Noe, Director of the National Museum of Health and Medicine, at the Armed Forces Institute of Pathology who graciously invited our Working Group to spend a memorable evening at the museum.

- Throughout our deliberations, J. Howell Smith, Ph.D., Chair, Emeritus, Department of History, Wake Forest University, has been of enormous help because of his wise and temperate advice and broad reaching knowledge of the field. His has been a steady hand for support of both Drs. Link and Toole, in all aspects of this undertaking.

- Edwin M. Yoder, Jr., D. Litt., who edited the Recommendations and Commentaries bringing his elegant prose style to our efforts.

- Steven Hochman, Ph.D., coordinated the Carter Center meeting and made certain that all of its facilities were available for ensuring a good beginning to our embryonic effort.

- Professor Miles Foy, J.D., of the Wake Forest University Law School, coordinated the conference at Wake Forest and on behalf of our group we express our special thanks to him.

CONVENERS

James F. Toole, M.D. and Arthur S. Link, Ph.D.

The White House Conference Center

Planning Committee:

David A. Drachman, M.D.
Professor and Chair of the Department of Neurology at the University of Massachusetts

Joel K. Goldstein, J.D.
Assistant Professor of Law at the St. Louis School of Law

Eugene A. Hildreth, M.D.
President-Emeritus - American College of Physicians

E. Connie Mariano, M.D.
Senior White House Physician

Lt. William McGee
Administrator (Chief Operating Officer), White House Medical Unit, The White House

J. Howell Smith, Ph.D.
Chair, Emeritus, Department of History at the Wake Forest University

Jerry M. Wiener, M.D.
Leon Yochelson Professor and Chair of the Department of Psychiatry at the George Washington University Medical School

Edwin M. Yoder, Jr., D. Litt
Professor of Journalism and Humanities at the Washington and Lee University

Wake Forest University Reynolda Campus

Planning Committee:

H. Miles Foy, J.D.
*Associate Dean and Professor of Law
at the Wake Forest University School of Law*

Jack Fleer, Ph.D.
*Professor and Chair of Politics
at the Wake Forest University*

Katy Harriger, Ph.D.
*Associate Professor of Politics
at the Wake Forest University*

Mr. Wayne King
*Director of the Journalism Program
at the Wake Forest University*

J. Howell Smith, Ph.D.
*Chair, Emeritus, Department of History
at the Wake Forest University*

Robert Walsh, J.D.
*Dean and Professor of Law
at the Wake Forest University*

Frank B. Wood, Ph.D.
*Professor and Section Head of Neuropsychology
at the Wake Forest University*

The Carter Center of Emory University:

Advisors

H. Miles Foy, J.D.
Associate Dean and Professor of Law at the Wake Forest University School of Law

Steven H. Hochman, Ph.D.
Faculty Assistant to President Carter at the Carter Center of Emory University

Mr. Wayne King
Director of the Journalism Program at the Wake Forest University

Bert E. Park, M.D.
Neurosurgeon Southwest Missouri Neurosurgical Group, PC

J. Howell Smith, Ph.D.
Chair, Emeritus, Department of History at the Wake Forest University

Jack Whisnant, M.D.
Professor of Neurology at the Mayo Clinic and President of the American Academy of Neurology

SUBCOMMITTEES

The subcommittee reports were received, accepted, and discussed extensively during the proceedings of the Wake Forest and the White House Conferences. These will constitute a large measure of the transactions of the three conferences which will be published in a separate volume under the leadership of Editor Arthur S. Link.

Balancing Public Disclosure with Patient Confidentiality:

Mr. Wayne King, Chair
Herbert L. Abrams, M.D.
Hugh E. Evans, M.D.
Phil Fontanarosa, M.D.
Ms. Cheryl Mills
Robert S. Robins, Ph.D.
Edwin M. Yoder, Jr., D. Litt

Identifying Criteria for Disability and Impairment:

David A. Drachman, M.D., Chair
John A. Gergen, M.D.
Jerrold M. Post, M.D.
Jerry M. Wiener, M.D.
Frank B. Wood, Ph.D.

Consultants:

Martin Abeloff, M.D.
Joseph Tenenbaum, M.D.

Investigating Advantages and Disadvantages of Formalized, Standardized Contingency Plans for Administration in Cases of Disability:

Francis Kittredge, M.D., J.D., Chair
Robert J. Joynt, M.D.
Bert E. Park, M.D.
Teresa Roseborough, J.D.
Jack Whisnant, M.D.

Strengthening the Position of the Physician to the President and White House Medical Staff:

J. Howell Smith, Ph.D., Chair
Eugene A. Hildreth, M.D.
Burton J. Lee, M.D.
E. Connie Mariano, M.D.
Lawrence C. Mohr, M.D.
T. Jock Murray, M.D.

The Role of the Spouse in Determining Disability and Ensuring Presidential Health:

Katy J. Harriger, Ph.D., Chair
Joel K. Goldstein, J.D.
Daniel Ruge, M.D.

Elements of Contingency Planning for Presidential Disability:

Lawrence C. Mohr, M.D., Chair
Joel K. Goldstein, J.D.
Katy J. Harriger, Ph.D.
E. Connie Mariano, M.D.
Edwin M. Yoder, Jr., D. Litt

Subcommittee on Executive Summary: Conclusions and Recommendations

H. Miles Foy, J.D., Chair
Robert S. Robins, Ph.D.
Francis I. Kittredge, Jr., M.D., J.D.

Subcommittee on Physician to the President:

E. Connie Mariano, M.D., Chair
Jonathan E. Rhoads, M.D.
Bert E. Park, M.D.
Jerrold M. Post, M.D.